Clear Your Mind

Regain Focus and Declutter

Your Mental Space

I0456206

Table of Contents

an illegal act, irrespective whether it is done electronically or in print. The legality extends to creating a secondary or tertiary copy of the work or a recorded copy and is only allowed with express written consent of the Publisher. All additional rights are reserved.

The information in the following pages is broadly considered to be a truthful and accurate account of facts, and as such any inattention, use or misuse of the information in question by the reader will render any resulting actions solely under their purview. There are no scenarios in which the publisher or the original author of this work can be in any fashion deemed liable for any hardship or damages that may befall them after undertaking information described herein.

Additionally, the information found on the following pages is intended for informational purposes only and should thus be considered, universal. As befitting its nature, the information presented is without assurance regarding its continued validity or interim quality. Trademarks that mentioned are done without written consent and can in no way be considered an endorsement from the trademark holder.

Introduction

Congratulations on purchasing your personal copy of *Clear Your Mind: Regain Focus and Declutter Your Mental Space.* Thank you for doing so.

The following chapters are going to focus on how you can truly become the best version of yourself. In today's over-stimulated and fast-paced world, the mind can often become overwhelmed; perhaps, more easily than was possible in the past. If you often feel as if your mind is racing faster than you can keep up, it's important that you care for yourself in a timely manner. Otherwise, you run the risk of living a life that is full of insecurities and unnecessary anxieties. It's safe to say that no one wants to go through life like that.

Instead, wouldn't it be great if you were able to train your brain to slow down and focus? That's what this book is going to teach you. After reading this book, you'll no longer feel as if life has too many elements to it. You'll likely have a better grasp on how to complete tasks and form relationships that will leave you feeling nourished, fulfilled, and like a successful human being. This can all be accomplished without the use of medication or alteration of the mind with a prescription. The truth of the matter is that prescription medication often brings with it unwanted side effects. These side effects can sometimes end up hurting the mind rather than helping it. That is why this book will seek to inform you about how you can refocus the brain without the use of medication at all.

The final chapter of this book is going to discuss the many benefits that will come to you and your life when you commit yourself to developing a greater sense of mental clarity and space. The reality is that mental clutter not only influences the mind but it can also lead to physical manifestations as well. Even if you're still not completely convinced about how important clearing the mind is prior to reading the last chapter, that last chapter should truly translate why your mind's health is not something that should be ignored. After all, you're the one who is seeing the world from your brain's perspective. This means that if your brain feels bogged down or slow, all of your interactions and interpretations of reality are going to also feel similarly. Taking the time to clear your mind and develop strategies for success is extremely important, especially when it comes to the longevity of your mental health.

Chapter 1: What Mental Clutter Is and the Different Ways It Can Manifest

Before we get into discussing how to fix mental clutter, it's important that you are able to recognize what the different types are. This chapter is going to look at five different types of mental clutter that can generally end up causing the mind to lose its focus. These types of mental clutter include putting ourselves down through pessimistic inner monologues, worrying, fear, guilt, and regret. After reading this chapter, you should be able to easily determine what type of mental clutter predominantly consumes your mind. Keep in mind that for all of us, it's likely that multiple types of mental clutter currently find space in your mind. This is completely normal, and there is no reason to feel down on yourself if you come to find that all of these types of mental clutter sometimes sit inside of your brain.

Mental Clutter Type 1: Negative Monologue

It's likely that most of us have a voice that dictates information to us in our head. This should not be confused with the idea that we have "voices in our head." This type of voice is perhaps one that simply voices the thoughts that you're having in your head. It could be the voice that prompts you to say something during a conversation or the voice that tells you what it is you truly want in a given situation. This is the voice that might speak to you regarding how you look when you look in the mirror or the voice that speaks to you in terms of your self-esteem.

Self-talk, in general, can be either positive or negative. This type of monologue can either be done aloud or to ourselves; however, when self-talk is negative rather than positive, this can create a significant amount of mental clutter in our heads. When you tell yourself that a certain feat that you're trying to accomplish is impossible, the reality is that this type of conversation can actualize a situation where you end up failing.

On the other hand, if you are able to cultivate positive self-talk within yourself, the result could end up being the opposite. Instead of failing, you could thrive. Negative self-talk can often create a negative mental environment within ourselves. Some common signs of this type of negative mental environment include feelings of self-doubt, feelings of ugliness or feelings of inadequacy. If you can relate to these feelings, know that you're not alone. This is a rather prevalent type of mental clutter, and most people do not even realize that negative self-talk is occurring within themselves until they truly stop and think about it.

Mental Clutter Type 2: Worrying

In addition to negative self-talk, another type of mental clutter involves worrying. For some people, worrying can be chronic. Sure, everyone worries about certain things once in a while, but some people tend to worry more than others. For these types of people, worrying can become almost addictive or compulsive. For example, for these types of people, it might be difficult to recognize that there are some situations that are out of an individual's control. Not everything in life is predictable, and yet for some people, this fact can sometimes prove to be unbearable. The result is a cluttered, worried mind.

Another major reason why worrying can take up a lot of valuable mental space is that unpredictability means that the future is uncertain. As you're going to see, a large portion of this book is going to be focusing on how you can capture the present moment, and relinquish your mind from focusing too much on the past or on the future. Worrying is a prime example of the fact that mental clutter is often caused by anxieties that are beyond the control of the individual in question. By shifting the focus of the mind onto more positive aspects of life, it's possible to evade and eliminate large lumps of mental clutter build up.

Mental Clutter Type 3: Fear

Fear can also clutter or stunt the mind's ability to process information as efficiently as possible. If you've ever experienced feelings of fear in regard to a situation that you've never dealt with before or perhaps because of the loss of someone important in your life, then you're already well aware of the fact that sometimes fear can literally stop you in your tracks. It prevents an individual from being able to accomplish what should or needs to be done while also being able to potentially manipulate the brain during the process. If you as an individual allow fear to penetrate your mind to the point that it's preventing you from doing something, then it should be clear that fear is a major type of mental clutter that should be eliminated from your life.

Mental Clutter Type 4: Shame or Guilt

Shame or guilt typically manifests in the mind when we are not happy with the decisions that we've made. This idea becomes twofold when the decisions that we've made in the past have ended up hurting people whom we care about or people who have trusted us in some capacity. Guilt can take up a lot of space in an individual's mind when he or she is unable to let go of their poor choices. Instead of letting these poor decisions go and becoming learning lessons, people can sometimes cling to their feelings out of guilt or shame. This type of clinging fuels a situation where the individual allows their self-worth to become tarnished and allows low self-esteem to develop as well.

Additionally, shame or guilt can open an individual's mind up to a situation where negative self-talk can ensue. For example, if an individual feels shame or guilt about a situation that unfolded in the past, they can begin to become resentful or angry towards themselves. Once angry and resentful, this is where negative self-talk can begin to form and take hold of the mind. Being able to acknowledge feelings of guilt or shame is often the first step towards relinquishing the mind from guilt's grasp. Once you are able to recognize that these types of feelings exist within yourself, you can then work towards not just forgiving yourself, but also forming a more positive relationship with your psyche entirely.

Mental Clutter Type 5: Regret

The last type of mental clutter at which we are going to look is regret. It's important to realize that every single, self-defined, happy person in this world has more than likely done something that he or she has ended up regretting. Making bad decisions is just one unfortunate reality about being a human. It's not about the decision itself; rather, it's more about how you deal with these decisions when they do not end up with an outcome that's in your favour that truly matters. It's common for people to focus more on the outcome of a situation and less on what was learned from this single experience. Being human involves being able to objectively look at what went wrong and where you can improve; however, it's possible to become too caught up in the past event, rather than being optimistic about how you can go about improving in the future.

For all of the types of mental clutter that we have discussed in this chapter, there is a common thread that seems to run through all of them. This common thread can be best defined as an inability to let go. If you can identify with any of the types of mental clutter that we've discussed, there is a chance that you're sometimes too hard on yourself from a mental perspective. Sure, everyone knows that he or she could have done something differently or better in a given situation, but the ability to release yourself from that type of burden is truly essential if you ever want to find mental clarity. Hopefully, by reading about each type of mental clutter that the mind can get trapped in, you are already able to see how you currently nourish the mental clutter that is in your own individual mind.

Chapter 2: Triggers That Can Lead to an Overactive Mind

Now that we've gone over some of the biggest types of mental clutter that exist, we are now going to turn our attention to specific triggers that can lead to a more cluttered mind as well. Within this chapter, all of the triggers which we are going to look at can be identified as being categorized within the types of mental clutter that were discussed in chapter 1. After reading this chapter, you will have a much better understanding of how your interactions with certain daily stimuli can influence your mind's activity. Let's take a look at some of these potential trigger points now.

The News

For some people, the news can be a trigger point that can cause unnecessary worrying, stress or even guilt. These days, it can sometimes seem as if everything on the news is all about negativity, violence or controversy. If you're someone who is used to watching the nightly news, a great way to test and see if the news is a mental clutter trigger point for you is to watch it and keep track of how you feel afterwards. Either write how you're feeling down or you can even use your smartphone to record your feelings on its voice recorder. It's important to take note of any feelings that may arise that have to do with the types of mental clutter that were found in chapter 1. For example, if something on your local news channel causes you to feel unsafe because of a crime that was recently committed near you, this will cause you to feel a sense of worry. These are the types of triggers that you should be looking out for while you're watching the news.

Once you've taken note of your feelings after watching the news, the next step is to go a few days without watching it. Step back from the chaos that the news brings to your eyes and ears, and see how you feel. It's likely that you'll find that when you don't watch the news, your head is able to be just a little bit clearer. When you don't have to think about the chaos that is going on in another country or the chaos that is going on in politics, it can become truly freeing. Of course, this isn't to say that you should completely hide from current events that are happening in the world; however, by recognizing that the news can sometimes clutter the mind in unforeseen ways, you might be able to protect your mind against it when necessary.

Money

Another trigger point that many of us can agree on that causes a lot of mental clutter is money. Especially in the United States, the notion of the "American Dream" is something that many of us still strive to achieve on a daily basis. Whether you're a millennial who is just moving towards the job market or a middle-aged person who is looking to save for retirement, money is something that can cause a lot of worry, fear, and even regret. If you're someone who seems to be constantly thinking about money and how to get more of it, there are a few techniques that you can use that may help you to think less about something that is unavoidably essential once you become a self-sufficient adult:

1.   **Alter Your Mindset:** One of the first things that you can do when it comes to money and the amount that you have is to change the way you approach it. If you find that you're currently thinking about money from the perspective of someone who is anxious and worried about it, maybe it would be more beneficial to be grateful for the money that you do have. This doubt about money can also come from a place of low self-worth. If you believe that you're not someone who is capable of making a lot of money, how do you expect to succeed? You are fully capable of making enough money in order to be comfortable. This recognition starts with understanding that you are in fact worth the money that you could be making.

2.   **Quit Chasing That Cheddar:** If you're currently worried about money because you feel

like you never have any even if you have a means of making it, it's important to be upfront with yourself about where your money is going. After you recognize where it's going, for the most part, the next step is to figure out where you can cut costs in regard to this expense, wherever possible.

The Past

Another trigger for many of us is our past. Sometimes, our past is our only reference point as we move through the complications of life; however, this does not mean that we should allow the past to define our future. When you tend to focus on the past, it can seem as if all of your inner demons shine brighter than they should. We've all made mistakes, taken others for granted, and have done things that were not smart in hindsight. When you focus on the negative aspects of your past, rather than on the positives, it's more likely to live in a present where you're overly hard on yourself. If you are someone who is often triggered by your past, there are a few questions to which you can resort to that will likely ease the tension that this type of thinking causes:

1. Are the circumstances of my past applicable to my current situation?

2. Am I overreacting?

3. Was the event in my past truly in my control?

These questions should be able to help you to walk away from stressful sensations that may occur in the mind that relate to the past. If you can begin to think about the past as being less defining to who you are today, it may lead to less clutter when you're making decisions in relation to the present moment.

Your Current Habits

If you live in something for long enough, it can seem like that's all there is. It's natural to get stuck in your current ways, even if these circumstances do not make you feel particularly happy. If you feel as if you have an attitude that goes something along the lines of, "Well, I can't change this, it's just the way that it is," then know that this is a great place to start when it comes to altering your perception of the world. If you think that your current circumstances are causing a significant level of mental clutter in your head, there are a few areas of your life that you can think about altering:

1.   **Your Associations:** We're going to get more into understanding the pillars of any sound relationship later in the book, but the people with whom you associate can often cause you to cultivate certain habits and ways of living. If these habits are not positive or make you feel bad about yourself, then it may be that these very people need to leave your life. This is a harsh reality to face, but it may be necessary.

2.   **Your Things:** Maybe, instead of constantly having to worry about money, you have plenty of it. Instead, you worry about the material possessions that you own. If you find that you equate happiness with the number of things that you own, you may also find that these things do not bring you happiness for the long-term. It might be time to reevaluate your

relationship with your things.

3.   **Your Job:** Your habits certainly include the current job that you have. Does your job bring you a sense of fulfillment and happiness? Or are you constantly thinking about how much you dislike your job and the people with whom you work? Even if you may currently think that it's completely insurmountable to leave your current place of employment, know that this is an obstacle that you're creating in your own head. Begin thinking about the career path of your dreams, and then take the concrete steps to get there in a timely manner.

Chapter 3: The Limiting Nature of Thinking Too Much

Now that you should have a comprehensive understanding of how your daily interactions with the things around you might be affecting your mental clutter, we are now going to focus on the problems that can occur when there is too much going on in your head. Of course, this chapter is not meant to scare you or make you think that you're doomed if you have too much mental clutter; instead, it's meant to enlighten you and encourage you to move forward. After reading this chapter, you will have a better understanding of how detrimental a life of clutter can be for the brain.

More Room for Error

Have you ever noticed that when you have a bunch of different thoughts on your mind, you have a more difficult time completing the task that is directly in front of you? This tendency is not simply a coincidence. In fact, it's been proven that the more brain activity that is occurring during a given period of time, the more likely it is for people to make mistakes. For example, let's say that you have a big final exam coming up for a class that you're taking, but you have a lot of other stuff going on as well. Your parents are getting a divorce, you think that your girlfriend is going to break up with you, and you're also having problems with one friend in particular. The final exam is where your focus truly needs to be, but you're finding that your brain is being constantly clouded by these other problems that are occurring in your life.

When this happens, it's best to take a step back. Try to look at your life objectively, rather than emotionally. I know that this concept can be easier said than done, but if you're able to look at things from a lens that is less invested in what's going on around you, you may find that you're able to focus on what needs your full attention more efficiently. While this may be difficult to do at first, if you practice focusing on something with your full attention, you're likely going to find that concentrating will become a little bit more effortless. In time, this ability to focus on one aspect of your life at a time could result in more success and less uncertainty.

Over complication

Another reason why decluttering the mind is so important is because when there is a lot going on in our brains, we tend to overcomplicate certain aspects of our life. When there are many different factors all coming together and happening at once, it's common for an individual to become nervous or overwhelmed by whatever is going on. Another common thing that happens when you overcomplicate a situation due to mental clutter is that the future can seem unbearable or stressful. This is because the complicated nature of your mind is drawing up potential outcomes that could occur. Spinning out of control, this causes you to feel out of control and alone. If you can, it's best to recognize when you're overcomplicating a situation. Slow down, and become aware of the fact that baby steps are often the way to lead yourself to a favourable outcome.

Thinking is Not Action

When you think too much, it can be stifling. If you're constantly planning for the future, there's a chance that you're actually never going to act on the plan that you're creating for yourself. Especially when there is too much going on in the brain, our thought process can sometimes feel like it's in a constant loop that won't stop. When this happens, it can become incredibly frustrating to attempt to even perform the smallest actions. If all those extra thoughts in the mind could clear, you'd be able to see more fully what needed to be done. It's this clutter that stops our ability to move forward and execute a plan that is both efficient and straightforward.

You Can't See

Of course, you're not physically blind when there is a lot of mental clutter taking up space in your brain; however, you are sometimes blind to fully seeing the world around you. For example, think of a particular chore that you simply hate to do. When you perform this chore, it's likely that you dread doing it the entire time that it's occurring. You may spend your time thinking about how stupid the chore is or how someone else should be doing it instead of you, rather than focusing all of your energy on the chore at hand.

For example, I hate to do laundry. I used to think of doing laundry as tiring, tedious, and dumb. These days, I try to think of doing laundry in a more positive light. Rather than thinking about everything that I hate about doing laundry, I try to think to focus all of my energy on the task itself. When I'm folding clothes, I concentrate on noticing what I'm actually folding. I look at the tags on the clothes and look at where they were originally made. I think about how I can perfect my folding technique to make my clothes look like they're in a retail store. It's these types of thoughts that make folding clothing more bearable for me, and these thoughts also allow me to truly take a vested interest in the task at hand.

Fear of Trying New Things

When you have too much going on in your mind, there's really no limit to the types of thoughts that you're probably having. The past, the present and even thoughts about the future are all tangled into one another and can be difficult to separate from each other at times. These thoughts can cause us to be fearful of trying new things that present themselves to us, especially if we are too hard on ourselves about how we handled something in the past. This fear of trying new things often comes from a fear of the unknown. While the cluttered mind can plan and attempt to anticipate what's to come, something that is completely new or unforeseen can seem unbearable or unimaginable. Wouldn't it be wonderful if you could simply look at new obstacles in your life with a feeling of excitement and courage? When you're able to clear the mind of clutter, a greater awareness of life's vast possibilities opens up and fear of the unknown becomes obsolete.

It's Exhausting

Lastly, another reason why mind clutter can feel limiting is that of its exhaustive qualities. If you've ever taken an important test or have been grilled at a pivotal meeting, then you know that thinking can truly be tiring. Did you know that you're burning your body's energy when you're thinking? It's the same as exercising, just for a different part of the body. In fact, scientists have gone so far as to prove that overthinking actually leads to a decline in glucose in the brain. Glucose, a form of sugar, is the body's primary source of energy. This means that when you're overthinking, you're actually wasting precious bodily energy. Think about the many things this energy could be better spent doing. Not to mention the fact that being constantly tired can lead to overeating, depression, anger, and a host of other issues. Why would you make yourself more tired if you didn't have to?

After reading about all of the various reasons why mental clutter can be limiting to your life, it should be even more obvious that you could certainly benefit from having fewer thoughts running through your head. When you have less to think about, you're able to truly expand not just your brain's ability to process information, but also expand your ability to experience life to its fullest extent. Thoughts are exactly that, just thoughts. Unless you are able to act on the thoughts that are running through your head, there's little reason to be thinking about the "what ifs" or the "maybes" in regard to situational outcomes. By thinking less about the infinite possibilities, you'll always be better off focusing on what's in front of you during any given moment of time and consciousness.

Chapter 4: Ways That You Can Clear All That Clutter

Speaking of taking action, what good would this book be if it couldn't provide you with some advice on how to clear some of the clutter that currently exists in your brain? This next chapter is going to discuss small things that you can do on a daily basis in an attempt to pacify and control the thoughts that could be bombarding your brain at any given period of time. After reading this chapter, you will have concrete courses of action that you can resort to if and when you find yourself in a situation where you're feeling overwhelmed by thinking too much. Let's take a look at some of these tactics now.

Mind Declutter Tip 1: Breathe

Whenever you're feeling overwhelmed, a great tactic is to simply focus on breathing. Close your eyes, and think to yourself, "inhale" as you inhale, and "exhale" as you exhale. By doing this, it will allow you to regain a feeling of control, at least within your own body. Deep breathing has been known to lower stress levels and blood pressure levels. In addition to being able to calm the physical body, concentrating on your breathing can allow you to achieve a greater sense of focus. Noticing your breathing forces you to think about only one thing, and this can help to stop the other thoughts that are chaotically vying for space in your mind during a given period of time.

Mind Declutter Tip 2: Work Out

Another great way to clear the mind of any excess clutter is to go to the gym and work out in some other type of way. Not only does exercising allow you to focus on the energetic activity that you're performing, but it also changes the mind in some scientifically proven ways. For one, exercise increases the endorphin production in your brain. Endorphins can be best described as a secretion in your brain that is used to relax or calm the body. Other benefits of exercising can include the following:

1.   It can increase your self-esteem.

2.   It can help to ease feelings of depression or anxiety.

3.   It can help you to sleep better.

4.   It can provide you with an added sense of control of your life.

5.   It can improve your mood and make you more optimistic.

If you currently do not do much in terms of exercising, becoming more active might be exactly what you need in order for your mind to slow down. Exercising can be as simple as going for a walk around your neighbourhood or doing some push ups in your bedroom.

Mind Declutter Tip 3: Start Writing More Down

Another way that you can teach your brain to stop moving so fast is to write your many thoughts down. Of course, you don't need to write down your thoughts in a formal journal if you don't want to; however, getting a journal might be a good idea. If you have a place where you can regularly go in order to decrease the number of thoughts that you're having, then you're likely establishing positive habits that will lead to long-term change. For many people, once they write down their thoughts, they feel as if the weight of their brain's activity has been expelled from their mind. Some of the topics about which you can consider writing, if you plan on starting a journal, include the following:

- Steps that you can take in order to achieve a certain goal that you have

- A list of your current worries

- Details about a relationship that might be straining your mental energy

Remember, it's your journal. There are no rules for it except for the rules that you set.

Mind Declutter Tip 4: Read a Book

Another way to clear the mind is by reading a book. Of course, you want to make sure that it's a good book before you dedicate yourself to reading it, but reading a good book will allow you to escape from reality in a way that may not be possible otherwise. Yes, watching television or going to see a movie can offer a similar feeling of escapism; however, these avenues of entertainment often do not allow the mind to work as hard as reading a book requires. Additionally, a book can occupy your mind with details that a movie or a television show cannot express to the mind in the most straightforward way possible.

Mind Declutter Tip 5: Keep a List

If you find that you often don't overthink things like your relationships but instead find that you focus a lot of your attention on what you need to accomplish, you might be better off keeping a list for yourself. Simply write down all of the tasks that are consuming your brain on either your smartphone, the computer or on a piece of paper. These days, it's possible to have your list with you wherever you go, which should make any task-oriented worry feel a tad bit calmer. When you do this, you're definitely taking some clutter away from your brain because you know that you have all of your tasks already written down together in one place. This will also allow you to organize your tasks more efficiently. For example, if you were to organize your tasks in the order in which they needed to be completed, you would have a list at your disposal that was always up-to-date and accurate.

Mind Declutter Tip 6: Say No to Interruptions

If you're a parent, then you probably can relate to the fact that sometimes it seems like you can never get anything truly accomplished. Just as you're about to try and get something done for yourself, someone in your family needs something *right away*. There are other types of interruptions that can occur, even if you don't have children. Today, our cell phones can often be a big source of distractions, and can sometimes interfere with our ability to just get it done. Think about the potential interruptions that you have in your life currently, and then consider whether or not some of these interruptions could be dealt with at a later time or when you're ready to take them on without any other distractions.

Mind Declutter Tip 7: Quit Procrastinating

We're all busy people, and it's natural to want to put things off until the last minute, especially when there is a lot going on; however, if you're someone who currently tends to wait to do something out of laziness or because you just "don't feel like it," then know that this might be the source of some of your mental clutter. The simple fact of the matter is that completing tasks is good for the mind. Sure, you don't want to be constantly finishing tasks obsessively, but if you don't address the things that you need to get done in a timely manner, there's a chance that these same tasks will end up occupying space in your mind until they're finished.

Even if you don't think that you need to work on all of the types of mental clutter that these particular tips pertain to, it's more than likely that you can relate to at least one of them or a couple of them. If one particular tip is speaking to you more than the others, it would be a good idea to start with attempting to try that one before moving onto any others. Additionally, don't be afraid to experiment with the different tips that were presented in this chapter. There are no rules saying that you cannot alter these tips and make them work for you to the fullest extent possible. These tips are simply the ones that many other people also resort to when they're feeling like there is too much going on in their heads. The hope here is that the tips that many other people use will also be useful to your mind as well.

Chapter 5: Tips on How to Let Go of the Past

While the present can often plague our minds when we have a lot to do, the past can often take hold of our mental facilities when it comes to dealing with the people around us. Additionally, it's safe to say that we all have had negative things happen to us in the past that we wish we could forget. Life can sometimes leave the emotional body with scars, and then it's up to us as individuals to heal them in the best way possible. This chapter is going to discuss how you can let go of the past in the step-by-step fashion. Letting go of the past is important because when you don't let go of the past, it can dictate how you react to things in the future. Let's take a look at this multi-step process now.

Step 1 to Letting Go of the Past: Recognize Why Letting Go Is Important

Let's make up a situation where you were hurt by a friend in the past. You feel as if this person left a mark on you emotionally. Because of this situation that occurred in the past, you now feel as if you can't trust anyone. This general sense of distrust, while you believe is protecting you from anyone else ever hurting you, has actually limited your ability to form positive relationships with the people around you. You constantly go back to the situation where your friend hurt you, and you can't let it go. This, in turn, creates emotionally-driven mental clutter that dictates how you live your life. Who wants to be driven to act by a situation that is not even relevant anymore? I definitely do not want to be, and I can guess that you also do not want to be either.

This is why letting go of the past is important, and recognizing this fact is the first step when you're looking to let go of a negative scenario that occurred previously in your life. In this way, you can think about being able to let go of the past as being a positive thing for primarily yourself. To this end, thinking about some of the following aspects should be able to help you deal with any issues regarding your past:

1. **Letting Go of the Past Relieves You**

of a Burden: Carrying around the weight of something that has hurt you in the past can be emotionally tiring. By forgiving these circumstances, you're able to strengthen your own individual psyche.

2. **Letting Go of the Past Relieves You of Resentment:** It's important to understand that when you choose to let go, this does not mean that you necessarily have to mend your relationship with the person who hurt you. Instead, focus on letting go of your anger, sadness or pain. This will help you to become a better you, without having to focus on the other person at all (if you would rather not).

3. **Letting Go of the Past Can Bring You More Understanding:** Often, people initially try to cause pain in other people because they are hurting inside for some reason. If you can recognize this and find it in your heart to be compassionate to the person who hurt you, it might be easier to let go.

4. **Letting Go of the Past May Require You Forgiving Yourself:** When we hold onto

the past, there's a chance that we also blame ourselves for the circumstances that occurred. Similar to finding compassion for the person who hurt you, it's also incredibly important to find compassion in your heart for yourself. Relationships are complex. It's entirely possible that you could be both the victim and have some responsibility in the matter simultaneously; however, if you find that this is the case, then you need to take responsibility and move on. There's simply no sense in making yourself feel guilty over it.

Step 2 to Letting Go of the Past: Quit Playing the Victim

Sure, you know someone who has hurt you in the past. We all know someone who has hurt us in the past. The person who hurt you made a decision to do so, and that's on them. That was their choice. Similarly, you are choosing to dwell on it. That's your current choice. This may sound a bit harsh to hear, but the second step towards letting go of the past involves recognizing that you are making yourself a victim. This is an important step in letting go of the past not because playing the victim is a sign of weakness, but because playing the victim allows the person who caused you pain to have control over you in some manner. Instead of continuing this pattern of victim-playing, consider doing the following the next time your mind becomes consumed by pain from the past:

1.   Remind yourself that you're in the driver's seat. Don't allow your brain to dwell on negative thoughts about the past.

2.   Turn your brain's attention to something more positive. This can be as simple as thinking of something you're looking forward to or reminding yourself of something that brings joy to your mind. By doing this often, you'll get into the habit of refocusing from the past onto something either in the present or in the future.

Step 3 to Letting Go of the Past: Exercise the Brain with Optimistic Declarations

Once you've started to refocus the brain from the past onto the present, your work isn't over. The next step involved with letting go of the past requires that you work on your self-esteem. If you think about something negative that has happened in the past often enough, it's likely that your self-confidence has been negatively influenced by it. To counteract this by-product of holding onto the past, you should consider rehearsing optimistic declarations to yourself. Below you will find some mantras that you can write down, say to yourself in your head or even say aloud while in front of a mirror. Doing this will help to train your mind to see yourself as being as worthy of love and affection as you truly are:

1.   I am the engineer of my world. I construct my environment and decide what lives in it.

2.   All of the things I need to be successful are already at my disposal.

3.   I choose to be happy above all else.

Feel free to create any other optimistic declarations that you think will brighten your day just a little bit.

Step 4 to Letting Go of the Past: Say What You Feel

When we bottle our emotions up, the problems that are making us angry or upset do not simply disappear or evaporate into thin air. No, these emotions stay inside of our brains. They torment us, and what often ends up happening is we create scenarios in our heads because we never said anything to the person with whom we're upset. We don't know what the outcome would be if we simply stated our feelings in the moment, and this causes the mind to race with "what if" scenarios all day long. To change this habit, you have to force yourself to become more open about what you're feeling, exactly when you're feeling it. Not only will this help your mind be relieved of these anxious thoughts, but it will also allow you to be less resentful about a situation because you let your thoughts be known as soon as the situation arose.

Step 5 to Letting Go of the Past: Look to the Past for Positivity

Finally, the last step towards letting go of the past involves reorienting your relationship with it. Instead of looking at the past and only considering the negative things that it's led to, what if you instead looked to the past and sought out the good things that have come from it as well? At least at first, when you're in a mindset of only thinking about the problems of your past, it can seem almost impossible to look to the past in a positive light. Try to remind yourself of the good times the past has brought with it, and this will allow you to clear the negative aspects of your past from your mind.

Chapter 6: The Power of Positive Thinking

The previous chapter on the topic of letting go of the past can be a nice transition into this next chapter. As you have already learned, one of the tactics that you can use in order to relieve yourself of stress about the past involves thinking more positively. That's what this chapter is going to be all about. In addition to helping us heal in regard to our sometimes painful past, positive thinking can be truly transformative in multiple other ways. This chapter will provide you with some tips on how to start thinking more positively, as well as prove that positive thinking can improve your mental state in more ways than one.

Why is Positive Thinking Important?

Thinking positively does not simply make you feel happier or provide you with a more optimistic outlook. Of course, these two outcomes are both by-products of thinking positively; however, there are far more benefits than these. Positive thinking has now been linked to your brain's reward system and pleasure stimulus. What this means is that once your brain feels the pleasure that positive thinking or happiness brings to it, it is going to reward itself in the hope of receiving more of this type of feeling. In other words, positive thinking can have a snowball effect on the brain. Once you start thinking more positively, your brain is not going to want you to stop. Instead, it is going to entice the mind to keep thinking in this way, so that you can feel good more often.

The manifestations of being able to think more positively about your behaviour in regard to your interactions with the people you encounter include being generally more optimistic and entertaining to be with. No one wants to be around someone who seems to be moping through life. It's likely that if you know someone who does not seem very happy when you spend time with them, it could be because he or she could do more positive thinking. On the other hand, if you know someone who typically seems to be pretty upbeat, hopeful, and carefree, at least a portion of their positive outlook on life probably comes from how they think on a daily basis.

The Brain and Your Optimistic Thoughts

From a more scientific perspective, positive thinking has been proven to influence growth that takes place in the brain as well. Specifically, positive thinking has been linked to stimulating the growth of neuron connections in the brain. Of course, even if you're someone who does not typically think positively, these connections are still going to grow; however, when you think positively, these connections are going to grow at a faster rate than they otherwise would if you spend all of your time thinking about what could go wrong instead of thinking about what could go right. While this may not matter much to you right now, especially if you're young, it's important to note that as you get older, your brain's ability to grow these neural connections is inevitably going to slow down. This means that if you learn how to think more positively, your brain is likely going to function more efficiently over a longer period of time.

In addition to being able to motivate the growth of neural connections, two other benefits that positive thinking can provide your body and brain have to do with output and analysis. Thinking positively has been linked to bringing to the brain a greater ability to be alert and process thoughts more quickly. Along these same lines, it has also been linked with being able to solve complex problems with more ease and in less time. This makes sense. When we think negatively, it can sometimes seem like we are only thinking of a poor outcome in regard to a particular situation. When we think positively, we are more likely to be open to experiencing a variety of outcomes, and this allows the brain to think of broader scenarios when it comes to figuring out puzzles or riddles.

The Body and Your Optimistic Thoughts

While the jury is still out on exactly why this phenomenon occurs in the brain, there is also evidence to suggest that positive thinking can lead to a more efficient immune system as well. There are countless stories out there about how people have recovered and fought back from serious and potentially deadly illnesses such as the AIDS virus and cancer. For example, perhaps you have heard the story of a man with terminal cancer who decided that he was going to cure himself by watching funny movies. All day and night long this man would watch comedies and laugh himself to sleep. He had cancer, but he was still going to laugh. This man was able to eventually rid himself of cancer that was deemed deadly. This is just one example of how positive thinking can overcome a negative situation and in this case, save a man's life.

You Are What You Think

Another way to look at positive thinking involves recognizing that our thoughts can often lead us to action (or inaction). For someone who thinks positively, he or she may see the world to be a better place where they can achieve any opportunity that they may desire. On the other hand, for someone who tends to think more negatively, he or she may see the world as a place where their current circumstances are the only circumstances that they will ever achieve. While the positive thinker uses his or her positive thinking as a platform to take a leap and strive to achieve a dream, the negative thinker will use his or her negative thoughts as a limiting tool that really stunts any potential growth.

It's probable that you have seen negative thinkers in action at one point or another in your life. These people might be the exact same people that they were in high school or they may be unable to clearly see the potential that they possess. Everything is always in flux, always changing. This includes you. Take the time to understand that as a human, you are constantly evolving. To settle and think negatively when it comes to your personal growth is something that should be avoided whenever possible. This is why positive thinking is important because often people become their thoughts.

How to Become More Positive in Deed, Action, and Thought

Now that you should have a better understanding of why positive thinking is important from a health perspective, we are now going to turn our attention to how you can become someone who thinks more positively than negatively. Sure, some people seem to be born with a greater sense of positively than others, but this certainly does not mean that you can't teach yourself to become more positive. One of the first lessons to learn as someone who is an aspiring optimist is that optimists are not positive all the time. These people fully understand that being too positive could also be detrimental. Instead, positive thinkers are typically people who see both the good and the bad in a given situation, yet they choose to focus more of their energy on the good than the bad.

When you're trying to be more optimistic, this is a good place to start. It's important to understand the difference between someone who is blindly optimistic to the point of harm, and someone who is realistic about what could go wrong and what could go right. Finding this type of balance is important, especially for someone who may tend to think more negatively than positively at the present moment. Rather than going all out and trying to be as optimistic as possible, it might be a better idea to first recognize both the good and the bad in a particular situation, before consciously turning your focus on the positive aspects of the situation at hand.

Volunteer

Once you've been able to concretely discern the difference between being blindly optimistic and being realistic, you can then move forward with finding tangible ways to become more positive. A great way to do this is to volunteer. You can volunteer your time in a variety of ways. Even if you hate the idea of giving back to your community or doing something for someone else for free, you can still find a small way to volunteer your time. For example, you could opt to spend an hour of your time every month visiting with your grandmother or grandfather who you may not see that often. You can opt to volunteer at your local library, a food kitchen or another type of facility where there are many people existing on a lot less than you have.

Write Down What You're Grateful For

If volunteering is just not for you, another way to become more positive is to document everything for which you're thankful. You can do this every night before you go to bed or every morning before you get up. It might be a good idea to dedicate a notebook to this endeavour, but you don't even have to write these thoughts down if you don't want to, at least at first. Instead, you can simply think about four or five things that happened during the day that made you happy or contributed to you having a better day. When you do this, it's best to think only about the current day that it is or the previous day if you're doing this in the morning. This will train you to think more about the positive details of your life than the negative details, and will likely help you to see that your life has many wonderful aspects in it.

Be Kinder

Lastly, you can be kinder to the people around you. We all could be kinder if we really wanted to be. When you're trying to think more positively, creating an environment where you are doing kinder acts for the people around you may be just the thing that you need. Not only will doing kinder things allow you to see your world from a new perspective, but this will also make you reconsider how you live your life on a daily basis. Some of the ways that you can be kind on a daily basis that will change your everyday routine include the following:

1. Pay for someone's meal when you're at a restaurant.

2. Compliment two people once a day.

3. Seek out people who may need help in everyday situations. Open yourself to noticing

how you can help someone.

Hopefully, this chapter has been able to prove to you how important thinking positively can be. Thinking positively is important not just for your sanity, but can also improve your body from a health perspective. Additionally, sometimes people tend to think that medicine can help them achieve positivity and happiness in the most efficient way. Maybe this is due to the rise in the accessibility of prescription medication in recent years, but you should try the tactics that were presented in this chapter before you run to your doctor and beg for some pills. You have the power to change the way that you think. You and you alone. This knowledge should empower you to at least attempt to become happier in an organic way before looking to medication to meet this end.

Chapter 7: Tips on How to Improve Your Focus

In addition to learning how to think more positively, another way that you can regain control of your mind and limit the amount of mental clutter that enters your brain is to improve your focus. This chapter is going to discuss some of the biggest external factors that can lead to a lack of focus, and will also provide you with some tips you can use to make your focus better and more consistent. Wouldn't it be great if you were able to focus on just one thought at a time, instead of allowing multiple thoughts to cloud your mind and prevent you from being productive throughout the day? After reading this chapter, you will have the tools at your disposal to do exactly that.

Why Is Focus Important?

Having the ability to focus is an important tool that every successful person should learn to cultivate to some capacity. When you are focused, it is much more likely that you will be able to achieve these mental capabilities:

1.   Set goals based on your own desires and preferences.

2.   Make choices with more certainty, based on what you truly want and what your goals are.

3.   Be able to figure out the path to take that will lead you to what you want.

4.   Find greater motivation from daily tasks because you know you are working towards a larger goal.

In contrast to the way that mental clutter can stunt the brain from accomplishing predetermined and straightforward tasks, priming the brain to be able to focus on a given task that will lead to something great for yourself brings with it confidence, drive, and enthusiasm. This is what focus can bring to your life that mental clutter simply cannot. It's safe to say that we'd all like to be optimally focused on what's good and positive for ourselves if this was always possible. Unfortunately, sometimes the clutter in our brains or the stress of life makes it seem like focus is all but a pipe dream.

What Causes You to Lose Focus?

The first step towards being able to clear your mind and focus on just one aspect of your life at a time involves figuring out what is primarily making you lose your focus in the first place. For example, if you're someone who is a self-described "scatter brain," it's important to understand that there may be more going on than simply being the type of person who can't keep track of anything. When we go through life, losing our house keys or completely forgetting that a major project deadline is coming up at work, there can be another larger problem at play. Perhaps your relationships could be stronger or healthier with the people who are in your life or maybe a sick parent or relative has your mind subconsciously stressing even when you're not consciously thinking about it. If a lack of focus is something that you can relate with heavily, the first step to fixing it is to be honest with yourself about any significant stressors that are plaguing your life.

Along these same lines, sometimes stressors in our lives can seem so taxing that we end up convincing ourselves that it's "no big deal" or that we don't really care about the outcome. Even when you tell yourself inwardly that something doesn't matter to you, this does not mean that you're not emotionally invested. This is why it's important to truly sit down with yourself and take some time to think about whether or not there is anything in your life that's taking its toll on your mental capacities. If you skip this step, you will likely end up still experiencing a lack of focus, even if you take other measures to try and remedy your focus problem.

Habits That Lead to a Lack of Focus

In addition, feeling unfocused due to external stress, another reason why your mind can sometimes feel like it is impossible to truly focus, is that of habitual choices that you're making in your life. Some of these types of habits that you can easily change in order to see whether or not it will improve your current lack of focus include the following:

1.   **Eating Too Much Sugar:** Obviously, eating too much sugar has been linked to causing chronic problems such as diabetes, but the complications that sugar can cause when it comes to mental clutter can go beyond that as well. For example, it's recently been proven that too much sugar in the diet has been linked to an increased chance of developing Alzheimer's disease when you're older. If this proven fact does not show you that sugar can definitely have a negative impact on our brain's ability to focus and organize information, then I don't know what will.

2.   **Not Eating Enough Fat:** Yes, consuming too much fat can certainly cause obesity; however, it's becoming increasingly clear that not consuming enough fats is bad for the brain. Did you know that most of your brain is made up of fat? Based on these findings, some doctors now believe that the brain will consume

itself when it can't find the proper nutrients that it needs. Without fat, the brain cannot produce the chemicals necessary to properly operate the body. Instead of focusing on a diet that is low in fat, it might be a better idea to instead focus on a diet that is low in carbohydrates. Most carbohydrates, when they're broken down, turn into sugar. As we've already discussed, digesting too much sugar can become a problem for the brain, especially later on in life. Some foods that are full of healthy fats include the following: avocados, eggs, and organic meat.

3.   **Dehydration:** Another way that you can probably eliminate at least some of your mental clutter is by drinking more water. More than half of the American population is considered to be frequently dehydrated. Think about it, your brain is made up of mostly water. Of course, it needs water in order to function at its maximum capacity. Drink more water, and develop better habits when it comes to drinking more water.

Vitamins and Focus

If you're looking to regain control of your mind and be able to think more clearly, you may also want to try upping your intake of vitamins B12 and D. Vitamin B12 is what helps you to keep your memory sharp, and a lack of it can also lead to digestive problems in older people. Vitamin D can be absorbed by your skin from the sun. It is known for improving the mood and has even been linked to improving depressive states. If you can clear your mind just a little by taking a multivitamin on a daily basis, why wouldn't you?

As you can probably tell by now, mental clutter does have to do entirely with the brain alone. The brain's ability to focus and patiently take tasks on one thought at a time has to do with a variety of factors, including ones that have to do with how you fuel it and keep it energized. Sure, writing down your thoughts in a journal or talking to a professional can help you to clearly slow down your thoughts, but if you are not taking care of your body and fuelling it with what it needs, it's likely to experience some glitches. One of these glitches could include your ability to focus, which could be contributing to your feeling of having too many thoughts at once.

Chapter 8: Knowing the Signs of a Bad Relationship

Sometimes it's not the way that we treat our body, but rather the way in which we treat ourselves emotionally that can lead to an overactive brain. The way in which we interact with the people around us and choose to invest our emotional energy into can be draining and exhausting if we don't make good decisions. This chapter is going to document some of the signs that can indicate you've found yourself in a bad relationship of some type. The next chapter will go over some of the ways that you can steady yourself against becoming involved in a relationship that is bad for you. It will largely discuss what you can do to form positive relationships in your life for now as well as far into the future.

Bad Relationship Clue 1: You Sometimes Feel Guilted Into Doing Something

Manipulation is a tool that people can use as a way to get others to do things that they want. A major sign that you've found yourself in a bad relationship is if you often feel like the other person in the relationship is making you feel guilty as a way to get you to do something. If you feel like telling someone that you don't want to do something, only for them to turn around and try to coerce you into doing it for one reason or another, then it is likely that there is a guilt dynamic occurring in this particular relationship.

Bad Relationship Clue 2: Your Feelings Are Not Taken Seriously

If instead of feeling guilted into doing things you don't feel as if your feelings are ever accounted for and taken seriously, then this is a different yet still incredibly detrimental problem that could be leading to your cluttered mind. When you're in any type of relationship, you want the emotional communication to be as straightforward as possible. Sure, some people are more skilled at communicating effectively than others, but you should always be able to express yourself emotionally to the people who care about you without having to worry about being taken seriously. If you can hear someone with whom you're in a relationship saying something along the lines of, "Calm down, you're too emotional" or "Why are you so upset all the time?" then it's possible that you're being trained to keep your feelings to yourself. When you keep emotions to yourself, they build up in your brain out of frustration because you're not able to voice them. It's as simple as that.

Bad Relationship Clue 3: You Lack Trust in the Person

If you're in a relationship with someone and have a hard time finding it in yourself to trust them, then this could be a major source of the mental clutter you've been experiencing. Often, when we can't trust the people who are supposed to care about us the most, our minds begin to race whenever we're not with them. Not only does this cause unnecessary mental clutter, but it also can lead to feelings of neediness or clinging.

For example, if you are dating someone but don't feel as if you can trust them when you're not around them, then you're probably going to want to be with this person as much as you possibly can. When you're not with them, you're likely going to be wondering whether or not this person is truly doing what he or she told you. At the same time, you could also be allowing your mind to wonder about where this person is and if they're being truthful. None of these circumstances are pleasant ones.

Bad Relationship Clue 4: You Can't Be Yourself

If you find that you change aspects of yourself when you're around a particular person, then it's definitely time to think about moving away from the relationship in question. If you have to alter who you are in order to be with someone, then this means that your mind is spending a lot of time figuring out how you can adapt yourself to be a better fit. No one should have to do that. It should be the other way around. Truthfully, you should be surrounding yourself with people who love you for the person you are, rather than the person they want you to be. Don't waste your time trying to be someone you're not. This will prevent you from spending too much time worrying about whether or not you're adapting in a favourable or unfavourable way when you're around that particular person.

Bad Relationship Clue 5: You Feel Like You're Being Controlled

No one should ever tell you what to do, who to see or when you *have* to do anything. Unless you're under the age of eighteen years old, you are in charge of your own life. It's that simple. If you know someone who is frequently trying to implement rules into your life when it isn't their place to be writing the rulebook, then this is yet another sign that the relationship that you're in is not healthy. Sure, it's reasonable for a person's significant other to want the other person to be faithful, but this desire does not give anyone the right to browse through your cell phone secretly, tell you who you can and cannot be friends with or try to control the money that you're making. These are clear and easy signs that the relationship that you're in needs to end, but many people put up with these types of controlling issues for one reason or another.

Bad Relationship Clue 6: You're Often Put Down

If someone with whom you have a relationship tells you often that you're not good enough for one reason or another, then it is a clear sign that the relationship is not right for you. No one needs someone putting them down all the time, but sometimes this can be done rather subtly. Even if the person is not coming out and directly saying that you're not good enough for one reason or another, you should still be looking for someone better for yourself. No one deserves to be treated that way. It's important to realize that there is a difference between being told you're not good enough on a frequent basis and being told you're not good enough during a fight that you're having. If there is a clear problem going on within the relationship that is more along the lines of a fight and less along the lines of daily verbal abuse, then you may just be going through a rough patch in your relationship at this particular moment.

The signs of a bad relationship that were presented in this chapter were not put here to simply educate you on how a bad relationship can be defined. Rather, it's important that you take the information that was presented in this chapter and think about how any of these circumstances make you feel on a daily basis. All of these signs can lead to mental clutter in the form of unnecessary worrying, stress or anxiety. Even if the people who are causing this stress in your life are your family members, by recognizing their part in your mind's clutter, you might be able to slowly start distancing yourself from them or reorienting your relationship with this person in a way that is both healthier and fairer to you.

Chapter 9: Cultivating Healthy Relationships for the Long-Term

You might be thinking to yourself, "Okay, I know the signs that make up an unhealthy relationship, but now what?" This chapter is going to answer that type of question that you might have on your mind. After reading this chapter, you will understand all of the components that are necessary if you truly want a relationship to not only work but thrive. Hopefully, you will find that many of these features already exist within the relationships that you've cultivated; however, you may also find that you could do some work here or there. Learning how you can best identify and nourish healthy relationships will allow you to live with less on your mind.

A Healthy Relationship Is a Responsibility

What I mean when I say that a healthy relationship is a responsibility is that each person who is invested in a relationship must be willing to take responsibility for his or her own well-being. The single biggest pitfalls for an otherwise healthy relationship is one where one person in the relationship feels like the other person should be caring for the other person's sense of happiness. To put it in a different way, if your partner or loved one does not love themselves, then they may try to make you responsible for their own flaws that they do not like. In order for a healthy relationship to flourish, both parties in it must be able to understand that ultimately finding happiness should be their own endeavour. To put this responsibility on their partner or loved one is not just unfair, it's also rather irrational. Some great ways to cultivate emotional responsibility in any relationship include the following:

-       Stating your feelings as soon as you have a problem, rather than allowing them to bubble up inside of you.

-       Resisting the urge to judge yourself and communicating with your partner when you do feel as if you're being judgmental towards your own thoughts or feelings.

- Resisting the urge to turn to drugs or alcohol when the "going gets tough."

- Refusing to see the other person as a scapegoat for the emotions that are proving difficult to deal with.

A Healthy Relationship Is Compassionate

If you have already learned how to be kind and understanding with yourself, then learning how to be compassionate and empathetic towards someone you're in a relationship with is all the easier. Being compassionate involves respecting the other person's point of view, rather than trying to challenge it at every turn. When you're able to see where someone else is coming from, that's when true love can grow and flourish. If you are currently struggling with finding kindness towards a person with whom you have a relationship, you can try some of the following tactics in order to improve:

- **Think About Yourself Less:** It is certainly important to think about your own feelings when you're in a relationship; however, it is also possible to think about your own feelings too much. Remember, a relationship is a partnership of sorts. Even if it's not romantic, a healthy relationship still involves compromising when it comes to always getting what you want. Practice keeping this in mind, especially when the other person's feelings are at stake.

- **Be Patient:** So often, we are more apt to try and write a story about someone in our heads, rather than see reality for what it really is. For example, if someone lied to you for some reason, your initial reaction could be rather hasty. You could jump to conclusions and think to yourself, "This person is nothing but a liar. There is no reason to be in this relationship anymore. The end." Instead, it might be smarter to try and evaluate things when you're less angry.

A Healthy Relationship Is Affectionate

Another aspect of any healthy relationship involves being able to share your joy of life with the people around you. Typically, this joy and happiness will come from a place of happiness that you have first been able to create within yourself. As you can see, a major part of being happy in a relationship involves first being able to properly care for yourself. One great way to find inner happiness is to spend more time alone. This does not mean that you have to end a relationship so that you can get to know yourself better; however, people often become better acquainted with their own personalities when they're single rather than in a relationship. Even if you don't want to remove yourself from a relationship, you can still cultivate a greater sense of self by perhaps setting time aside for when you're either alone by yourself or choose to go out with friends when it does not include your significant other.

A Healthy Relationship Has Conflict

In a healthy relationship, conflict is not always about having giant screaming matches or having to be "right." Contrastingly, a healthy relationship is bound to go through ebbs and flows. In a healthy relationship, a conflict does not result in screaming (it can, but it doesn't *always* result in extreme fighting). It ultimately results in growth. By being able to understand where the other person is coming from, both people in the relationship are better able to communicate and come to a compromise. Additionally, successfully reconciling with conflict can help you to see that both people in the relationship are not solely motivated by a sense of needing control or dominance. This should also ease your mind a bit because you know that when conflict does arise, it is likely not going to be earth-shattering.

A Healthy Relationship Is the Ability to Share Joy in Success

If you find that you're currently in a relationship where the other person does not visibly show excitement when something good happens in your life, then this is a huge problem that should be addressed sooner rather than later. If the person with whom you're in a relationship can't see that your accomplishments should be celebrated and not ignored, then this is likely to hurt both your self-confidence and your psyche. If you do not currently feel as if a person who is in your life expresses happiness for you adequately, then this is something that you should look into changing. The best piece of advice here is to start by trying to change your own habits. Perhaps you don't get excited enough when something good happens in your partner's life, which is why he or she does not get too excited when something exciting happens to you. Perhaps, instead of being completely bad and wrong, there is simply a dynamic that needs to be altered here.

Similar to the previous chapter, the inability to integrate these concepts into your current relationships could very well result in more anxiety and less surety in your own mind and life. If you can communicate with your loved one and he or she is willing to go through the process of looking at your relationship through the lens that this chapter provided, then it's likely that you will end up learning more about your partner and more importantly more about yourself. This will also allow you to alleviate frustrations or anxieties that could be cluttering your mind on a day-to-day basis. It's likely that you have many other things that you could be worrying about. Your relationships do not have to be one of them.

Chapter 10: Tactics for Decreasing Anxiety Now

The term "anxiety" or "anxiety disorder" seems to be at an all-time high these days. Anxiety can definitely lead to large amounts of mental clutter, especially if the trigger for your anxiety has to do with your work life or your home life. There are many different types of pills and medications that are prescribed to people who have an excess of anxiety; however, there are plenty of remedies that you can attempt to turn to before immediately deciding that you need medication. With an even bigger rise in the health sector in the United States, it can even sometimes seem as if people are overmedicated and made to believe that they have problems related to anxiety that only medication will fix. Let's take a look at some of the signs that could infer that your mental clutter is being caused by anxiety, and then we'll look at some of the ways that you can remedy this without the use of medication.

Generalized Anxiety

A generalized anxiety disorder can be best defined as a disorder in which a person worries about life often without being prompted. Typical stress triggers include worrying about one's health, work, family, and money. You might be thinking to yourself, "I think I have a generalized anxiety disorder!" based on that definition; however, it's important to understand that these symptoms are identified as being particularly drastic when defined under the umbrella of generalized anxiety. This means that if you are anxious but it doesn't occur every day or doesn't occur unprompted, then you probably do not have what's known as generalized anxiety. It's important to understand this distinction because some doctors have been known to diagnose people, who do not have generalized anxiety, with this disorder. This can lead to the prescription of anxiety medication when it is not truly needed. Some symptoms of having a generalized anxiety disorder include the following:

-        Not being able to fall asleep

-        Physical muscle stiffness or tightness

-        An inability to ever find relaxation

-        Becoming tired very easily

-        Not being able to concentrate or feeling as if the mind is completely barren of thought

Remember, unless the symptoms that you're experiencing could be considered to be drastic or intense, you probably do not have an anxiety disorder; however, this does not mean that you do not experience anxiety on a higher-than-average basis.

How to Treat Your Anxiety at Home

Many of us are not interested in becoming potentially reliant on anxiety medication that our doctor could provide us; however, some people are. If you simply do not want to work through your anxiety naturally, then you should consider heading to your doctor and inquiring about how he or she can help you with anxiety. If you are interested in figuring out a way to deal with your anxiety organically, then keep reading. This section will look at some of the ways that people have learned to treat their anxiety on a daily basis.

Anxiety Remedy 1: Sleep More

A major culprit when it comes to an individual's increased sense of anxiety tends to be sleep. Yes, it would be great if we did not need to sleep in order to be on our "A" games all the time, but this is simply not the case. You probably already know that an adult should be providing themselves with around 8 hours of sleep every night, but you probably also know how infrequently we're able to find this amount of sleep. If you don't think you'll be able to find a way to sleep for 8 hours every evening, perhaps finding room for 20-minute naps throughout the day could even help you to become less anxious. A 20-minute nap (also known as a "power nap") will allow you to feel refreshed and rejuvenated, without causing you to feel as if you want to continue sleeping for the rest of the day. These smaller naps can truly come in handy if you're someone who frequently finds him or herself wishing that you'd gotten more sleep the night before. This type of nap is able to clear your head and allow you to regain more control over your thoughts.

Anxiety Remedy 2: Spend More Time with Friends

Social anxiety is another type of anxiety that can sometimes limit the amount that we're able to accomplish and do throughout the day. If you know that you're someone who tends to shy away from social gatherings because of the fear and anxiety that you feel in regard to these situations, it's important to understand that pushing yourself to attend these types of parties or outings is the only way that you'll ever be able to get over this. If you can't connect with others, you're probably going to end up feeling even worse if you stay home because you'll spend your whole time at home thinking about whether or not you should have gone. Remember, it's important to not allow your mental clutter to prevent you from taking action in life.

Anxiety Remedy 3: Become More Accepting of It

You shouldn't think of yourself as being in a war with your anxiety. For some people, leading a calm and uneventful lifestyle just isn't in the cards. Instead of giving in to your feelings of anxiety and the negative way that it makes your mind and body feel, you should instead think about your anxiety as something that you need to work on daily. No one said this was going to be easy, but if you can begin to change your perspective of your anxiety to be something that you can fix rather than something that is "wrong with you," then you are more likely to find success when it comes to this area of your life. As you can see, doing this will change your perspective and make it more positive. As we already know, thinking positively is a proven way to achieve greater mental strength and clarity in your life.

Anxiety Remedy 4: Put Yourself Out There More Often

As with many other aspects of our lives, there is an element of anxiety that has to do with practice. Think about it – can you currently imagine yourself being a stand-up comedian or an actor on a nation-wide television show? Just thinking about this type of pressure is enough for some people's hearts to start beating faster, but we also know that there are other people in the world who take on this type of stress with ease. This is because the comedians and the actors of the world spend their lives practicing standing in front of people telling jokes or acting out long scenes for entertainment purposes. As with anything else in life, the more you do something, the less scary it becomes. Anxiety works in largely the same way.

If there is a certain anxiety trigger that you know frightens you irrationally, then you should work towards pushing yourself to get over that fright and stress in some way. The best way to do this is to perform this activity anyway, even though you know it brings you stress. If you do this action often enough, you're going to find that it will likely become less stressful. It may even be a good idea to ask yourself the question, "What's the worst that could happen?" This will allow you to put into perspective what's scary to you, and how it is rather an irrational thought to have. This might ease your mind a bit.

Chapter 11: Activities That Will Lead to a Greater Sense of Calm

This book has loosely discussed the notion of how habits can change the way in which we interact with and view the world. This chapter is going to expand on that concept. We are going to be looking at various types of hobbies that you can invest your time in that can lead you to a calmer, mental state. If you invest your time in any of the activities that are presented in this chapter, you should be performing this activity *at least* once a week, if not more often. All of the activities, which we're going to look at, will be able to slow your brain down and help you to find some ease within the busyness of your everyday life.

Mind Decluttering Hobby 1: Doing Yoga

If you don't know much about yoga, then you may currently feel as if yoga is only for bendy and thin people who worry too much about the latest activist movement and being vegetarian. In contrast to popular conceptions of yoga, it does not have to be just for these types of people. At its core, yoga can lead to a state of mental clarity because it forces you to think about your body's movement, and this takes away your brain's ability to think about what is going on in your life during a given period of time. Yes, there are components of yoga that may be too "spiritual" for your taste, but you do not have to invest in these components of the practice at all. If you're worried or too shy to attend a formal yoga class, the best place to start looking into this hobby is on the internet. Simply type in "yoga class online free" and you're guaranteed to find a yoga video or two that can walk you through a basic yoga class.

Mind Decluttering Hobby 2: Listening to Music

It has been proven that listening to music can have a calming and relaxing influence on the mind. Some of the benefits of listening to music on a frequent basis include being able to decrease anxiety and even pain, instil feelings of empowerment, and improve your mental health as well. Additionally, some studies have found that the rhythm of music can stimulate the brain and alter its processes for the better. If you do not currently listen to music as a way to de-stress, this is a great hobby that you should consider doing with some headphones on a frequent basis.

Mind Decluttering Hobby 3: Gardening

Even if you're someone who does not consider themselves to have a green thumb, gardening can still be therapeutic for the mind nonetheless. Not only does gardening allow you to be outside in the sun (which allows you to get more vitamin D), but it also allows you to notice the details that are required when something needs to be nurtured and provided for in order to be able to live. Additionally, there are scientific studies that have been done suggesting that the bacteria that can be found in plant soil stimulates the serotonin centres in our brain.

Serotonin is a chemical that is released in the brain that makes you feel more attentive, less stressed, happier, and generally more pleasant.

Mind Decluttering Hobby 4: Taking Photos

If you've ever been interested in trying photography, but have not invested any energy into it for one reason or another, know that photography can be incredibly calming for the mind. Taking photographs forces you to notice the details of everyday life. When you take photographs, you get to be an invisible witness into intricacies that you may not be able to notice otherwise. Of course, photography can end up being an expensive hobby, but it doesn't have to be. While you may not want to exclusively use your smartphone to take photographs, you can find a cheap enough camera for a couple of hundred dollars. Even if your camera isn't the nicest, the act of taking photographs can allow you to see the world in a new and invigorating light.

Mind Decluttering Hobby 5: Doing DIY Projects

Another way to bring the mind to a place where it's forced to focus on smaller details is to invest your time into doing DIY (Do It Yourself) projects. These projects can be especially enticing if you own a home and are looking to improve the look of your home on the cheap. These days, it seems as if all you have to do is Google the DIY project you're interested in doing, and more than likely someone has provided information about how to do it on the internet. From a scientific perspective, studies have shown that doing small projects on your own can lead to your brain aging more slowly. This has to do with the problem-solving nature of these types of projects.

Mind Decluttering Hobby 6: Knitting

Similar to doing DIY projects, learning how to knit or crochet can also be great for the brain. Specifically, knitting requires that you move in a repetitious pattern. This type of activity where you are continuously doing the same motion over and over again has been proven to be able to stimulate the parasympathetic nervous system. The parasympathetic nervous system is responsible for decreasing the body's blood pressure and can be considered to be the opposite of the sympathetic nervous system. The sympathetic nervous system is the one that is responsible for the body's "fight or flight" response. This means that when you perform the action of knitting, you are countering the effects on the body that can be caused by stress. Who knew that an activity that's typically associated with old ladies could be so calming?

Mind Decluttering Hobby 7: Painting or Drawing

Sure, not everyone is gifted with a paintbrush, but it has been proven that even doodling in a notebook can lead to better concentration in the classroom. These days, you have a few options when it comes to wanting to paint or draw. First, you could choose to buy yourself a canvas and some paint and paint along with the notorious Bob Ross. The late painter's television show can be found on Netflix, and Ross makes it easy to follow along and paint with him. Because it's on Netflix, you can even pause the show whenever you want in order to ensure that you're following the directions correctly.

Another option that you have, if you're not at all confident of your painting skills, is to instead invest some of your money into those infamous adult colouring books. While these books may seem a tad cheesy, their effect on the mind should not be taken for granted. Similar to knitting, these colouring books often entice you to find patterns within the shapes that you can colour similarly. The patterned nature of these designs allows the brain to relax and direct its attention more fully on the activity that you're performing.

You should try to integrate at least one of the hobbies that were presented in this chapter into your weekly routine. Once you start doing one or a multiple of these activities with more frequency, you're more than likely going to find that you do feel calmer and can think with more clarity throughout the week. Additionally, none of the activities that were presented in this chapter demand much in the form of time from you. Instead, you have the freedom to engage in these activities as much as or as little as you'd like.

Chapter 12: Social Media and Its Effects on Our Psyche

While the hobbies that were presented in the previous chapter can provide you with more feelings of positivity and less mental clutter, there is a different type of hobby that almost everyone who lives in the modern age can agree they would be better off with less of. This hobby is the hobby of surfing social media networks. This chapter is going to look at what social media can do to the brain in the form of stress, and why it might be a good idea to turn your back on social media, at least every once in a while.

Social Media – What Are the Risks?

If you think that social media does not have the power to take hold of your mental clutter and amplify it significantly, think again. A major aspect of social media has to do with pictures. These pictures are often of people taking "selfies" but they can also portray the fact that individuals are living extravagant lives that are extraordinary in nature and perhaps unlike your own. For example, let's say that you have a friend who is always traveling and this person takes photos of themselves in beautiful places all around the world. You're happy for your friend, but at the same time, you know that you yourself do not have the same opportunities as this person.

Seeing these types of things on any social media platform can lead to a feeling that is commonly known as "FOMO" or Fear of Missing Out. This is a form of stress. You'll know that you're experiencing FOMO if something on social media causes you to think to yourself, "How can I get more money? Why isn't my life like that?" and "What does this person do that I don't?" These types of feelings can become common and almost normal to experience these days because we are so used to allowing social media to take hold of our psyches. Many people have come to fully identify with their social media accounts, perhaps even more than they are able to associate with their personas in real life. This too can become a problem because it puts more stress on the brain to try and please two different platforms of reality simultaneously.

Curation Nation

It's also important to understand that if you do find yourself becoming jealous while you're looking at someone's social media account for one reason or another, you could be jealous about something that is not even entirely real. Some people place so much emphasis on their social media accounts that they end up spending more time worrying about that than they do their actual lives. For example, perhaps you know people who literally spend a few hours taking photos for their social media accounts. After they take the photos, they spend just as much time editing their photos in Photoshop so that they can look just right, before posting them to their social media profile.

You might be thinking to yourself that this type of behaviour seems incredibly outlandish or unlikely, but I promise you that there are plenty of people out there who act in this manner. This means that their social media profiles are not even a true reflection of their lives or themselves. By editing the photos to no end, they are curating a life that is a tad fictitious in nature. If you ever find that you feel as if social media is bringing you down, one of the first things that you can do is remind yourself of this fact.

Social Media Shows You the Stress of Others

In addition to bringing you more anxiety and mental clutter due to the jealousy that social media can create for a person, another problem with social media is that it opens you up to other people's stress. For example, users of the social media platform Facebook are able to see anything that their friends post as soon as they log onto the site. What this means is that it's possible for you to be bombarded with stressful information constantly. If your friend's mom is going to be having gastric bypass surgery in a few days, she might ask you to pray for her mother. If your other friend's husband is going through cancer and she posts about how difficult it's been, you're going to have to read it. These messages can connect us, sure, but negative information can also plague us and stress us out the same way that these negative events are affecting the people we're friends with on the Facebook platform.

What to Do When Social Media Is Causing Mental Clutter

Now that we've discussed some of the things that social media can do to our minds, let's turn to what you can do if you'd like to decrease the mental clutter that social media is bringing to your life. One option that you have is to delete all of your social media accounts from your phone. This will allow you to only be able to access your social media accounts while you're in front of an actual computer. Obviously, this might not make much of a difference if you're on a computer all day long, but if you're not in front of a computer every day, then this could have a major impact on the amount of time that you spend on social media.

Choose to Disengage

Another option that you have is to delete one or multiple social media accounts that you currently have. Before you do this, it's important that you check in with yourself and see how each form of social media makes you feel from a mental perspective. For example, if Facebook makes you feel as if you're missing out on something or you feel a lot of anxiety whenever someone posts something political, these could both be reasons to consider deleting your profile. On the other hand, if you do sometimes find yourself feeling anxiety over the scenarios mentioned above, but also know that Facebook is able to keep you connected with the friends that you have all over the world, then you may want to sacrifice your feelings a bit in the pursuit of maintaining important friendships.

Choose One Day of the Week to Fully Unplug

Another, perhaps more practical, way to distance yourself from any tension that social media sometimes can cause you is to choose one day of the week that you dedicate to not going on social media at all. This can include your email as well if you'd like because email is also a technological tool that can often lead to high levels of stress. While it may initially be difficult to separate yourself from your social media profiles for an entire day, you may come to find that you look forward to the day of the week that you chose. It could also become easier than you think to unplug yourself from the internet for at least one day out of the week. This way, you don't have to completely delete any account, but you're also able to distance yourself from the thoughts that social media can cause.

There's an App for That

Lastly, below you will find a list of apps that can help you to unplug. All of them vary a bit in how they're used, but they are all essentially designed to prevent you from being able to access the apps on your phone throughout the day:

1.   Offtime
2.   BreakFree
3.   Flipd

4.   AppDetox

5.   Moment

Chapter 13: Tips on Meditating

Moving away from social media, we are now going to focus our attention on a completely different subject. This chapter is going to focus on the process of meditating, in the hope that you can begin to develop a sound meditation practice. You don't have to be a guru or a hippie in order to become a person who meditates. As you're going to find, there are many scientific benefits that meditation provides for the body, and many of these benefits directly relate to the pursuit of having less mental clutter in the head. Let's take a look at what these benefits are, as well as the steps that you can take to start meditating as soon as possible.

What Is Meditation?

Essentially, meditation is a technique that some people use as a way to slow down the mind and figure out exactly how they are feeling during a particular period of time. Some people have a meditation practice that requires them to meditate at least once a day while many other people are less strict in their meditative ways. The point of meditation is to be able to slow the mind to a point where you begin to see reality for what it truly is. What that means is that instead of looking at a situation in your life through a primarily emotional lens, you're able to instead look at a situation with more objectivity and rationale. This translates to eventually being able to see situations more objectively when you're dealing with something. Do you ever feel like you're too emotional when you find yourself becoming angry or upset with someone? These are the types of emotions that meditating can help you to deal with in a more rational and less impulsive manner. When you begin to meditate, you open yourself up to understanding how to become humbler and less reliant on the identity that you've created for others to see.

Meditation and Mantras

A major concept that has to do with meditation is the notion of a mantra. Mantras can be best described as sayings that are repeated over and over in your head during a meditation practice. Mantras are not essential when you're meditating; however, they can be incredibly helpful when you're looking to find the concentration. For example, an extremely simple mantra that can be used when you're first beginning to meditate is to inhale and think, "Let" and exhale and think "go." The point of a mantra is to be able to repeat something over and over again to the point that you don't have any other thoughts. This allows the brain to slow down, and that is when meditation can truly begin.

It's also important to understand that even if you decide to meditate for a certain period of time and can't get your mind to concentrate on your mantra, this does not mean that your meditation practice for the day was a failure. Spending anytime alone, even attempting to meditate, is always going to be a successful meditation practice. Think about it – we live in a society where our brains are constantly being bombarded by information and stimuli. Be it advertisements, television shows or miscellaneous internet content, our brains hardly ever have the chance to just sit there without interruption. This is why meditation is important, and why there is no "bad" meditation practice. It makes sense that your brain would sometimes be unwilling to conform to a state of stillness. It's not used to it!

The Benefits of Meditation

I could write an entirely different book solely on the benefits that meditation can provide your life. Some of these benefits include the following:

1. Meditation can decrease depression: Some scientists believe that meditation can be ever more successful in treating depression than can antidepressant drugs.

2. Meditation can aid in the reduction of anxiety disorders in people: Again, it has been suggested that meditation can cure anxiety disorders better than medication can.

3. Meditation increases the brain's grey matter: Grey matter in the brain allows the brain to concentrate more effectively and control your emotions more efficiently.

How to Meditate

Meditating is fairly easy to perform. In fact, even after you read this section, you can adapt these instructions if you'd like to better adhere to your preferences or personal meditation style.

Step 1 for Meditation: Find a Quiet and Clean Space

It's safe to say that only people who have been meditating for years are able to meditate in a location that is bustling with people or distractions. You need to find a quiet and respectable space where you can meditate. What this means is that this space should also be quiet as well as clean.

Step 2 for Meditation: Find a Comfortable Seat

Regardless of whether you plan on meditating for two minutes or two hours before you begin, you need to make sure that you have a comfortable seat. This is important because once you begin to meditate, you want to make sure that you're not going to move from the position that you're in. A great way to meditate is to sit cross-legged on the floor, making sure that your back is extremely straight; however, you can also choose to meditate in a chair that has a back. I've also meditated lying down, but this does not always work for everyone.

Step 3 for Meditation: Close the Eyes and Acknowledge Your Thoughts

Once you have a comfortable seat, begin to close your eyes. You'll already know from closing your eyes to fall asleep that just because you close your eyes, this does not mean that your thoughts are going to stop. From here, simply begin to notice what you're thinking about. The ultimate goal is to be able to notice the thoughts that are coming to you, but try and let them pass. This can be seen as being similar to things that are going by on a conveyor belt. They're not necessarily going to stop, but they're not going to stop moving and require attention either.

Step 4 for Meditation: Begin Practicing Your Mantra

Once you've established a distant relationship with your active thoughts, the next step is to start practicing your mantra. On your inhale, you think the first portion of your mantra, and on the exhale, you think the second portion of your mantra. You can be creative with your mantra; it does not have to simply be "Let go." It can relate to anything in your life that you'd like to work on, such as, "Do not settle" or "You are beautiful."

Plan a length of time to meditate prior to starting. Set a timer for yourself, and then set your phone aside. Remember, it's important to not be too hard on yourself when it comes to meditating. It might be difficult to train the mind to concentrate on nothing, but it's well worth the effort. If you're consistent, there's no doubt that you're going to see an improvement in how your brain reacts to stressful and anxiety-ridden situations. Stay disciplined, and remember that it typically takes about two weeks for any habit to truly stick.

Chapter 14: How Mess Can Lead to Stress

If you've ever seen the television show called *Hoarders*, then maybe you can already agree with the idea that clutter can certainly cause the brain to feel overwhelmed and anxious. Simply watching that television show where people are living amongst far too many things is enough to make any rational person want to go to that person's house and help them start cleaning up. This feeling of increased anxiety when things are messy is one that can be described as normal. This chapter is going to look at how mess can lead to stress from a mental perspective, and what you can do to prevent yourself from feeling this way when a mess does arise.

Why Is Clutter So Darn Stressful?

While we all know that clutter can indeed lead to stress, less of us know why that is. Clutter can cause stress for a few reasons, which we will look at below:

1.   **Clutter can slow us down:** When we need to find something quickly, clutter prevents us from being able to do that as quickly as possible.

2.   **Clutter stunts creativity:** When your environment is cluttered, your brain actually feels less inclined to think creatively and solve problems. It's as if your brain can feel the lack of physical space in a room and is responding to it.

3.   **Clutter is lonely:** When your living space is cluttered, it can make you embarrassed to have other people come over and share your space. This can lead to isolating ourselves or closing ourselves off from the people around us, which is never a good thing.

4.   **Clutter is a list that never ends:** When there's stuff everywhere, it's as if our brain is always turned on. To our minds, we always have something to do that will eventually (hopefully) lead to less clutter. This can be exhausting for the mind.

5.   **Clutter leads to never being able to relax:** Because of the fact that our brains are

constantly working to deal with the mess in our homes or our immediate environment, it makes it harder to relax. Even when we're watching television or taking a nap, part of our brain is still trying to coerce us into cleaning up our mess.

6.   **Clutter is distracting:** When there's so much that's physically in our way, it can be limiting for our brain to think clearly. Clutter can truly be equated to being similar to the clutter that's in your head when there's a lot going on. How are you supposed to focus on just one thing at a time?

As you can see, clutter should not really be considered benign or something that has no consequences for the brain. Clutter in your physical environment can lead to increased clutter in your head. If you're someone who has an incredibly messy space at home, then a relatively simple way to begin working towards a clearer head is to clean your space up. Let's take a look at a few other ways you can fix a cluttered environment:

1. **Never Leave Your Work Area Messy:** If you don't want to even begin to think about decluttering your home, you can begin by attempting to declutter your workspace every day before you go home. This will allow you to feel fresh and ready to work as soon as you get to your office or wherever it is that you do work.

2. **Clean Up Papers Frequently:** The amount of junk mail that we receive from the mailman can truly be surprising. If you're like me, you might have the tendency to leave your junk mail lying in a pile somewhere for an extended period of time. Stop this behaviour.

Go through your mail as soon as you get it, and throw away your junk mail right away.

3. **Give All of Your Things a Home:** Everything in your living space should have a home. It's that simple. As soon as you remove a thing from its home in your living space, it needs to go back to its home when you're finished. Being strict and implementing this type of rule into your life will lead to a cleaner home.

4. **Do You Really Use It?** Look around your home and identify the things that you do not actually use. We all are guilty of holding onto our physical things for the wrong reasons. Go through each area of your home, and take an inventory of the things that are excessive or haven't been used in years. Ask yourself: why are you holding onto this particular thing? If you can't come up with a good reason why you're holding onto it, then get rid of it.

5. **Perform One Decluttering Activity Once a Day:** Finally, if you truly want to declutter the physical space around you, you should seek to perform one decluttering action

once a day. This action can be large or small, but the ultimate goal should be to slowly work towards a space that is completely clutter-free. Even if one day your decluttering activity consists of making a plan of how you're going to better organize your physical space, that still counts. One day, you'll look around, and the clutter will have been cleared.

Hopefully, this chapter has been able to prove to you that physical clutter can directly lead to a situation where your brain feels a lot more cluttered as well. Now that you've read this chapter, you should have both the reasons why decluttering your environment is important, along with steps that you can take in order to declutter your space now. Start by clearing your space based on one of the tactics that was presented in this chapter, and see how you feel. Sure, the work involved may be difficult, but it's well worth it, especially when your brain's clarity is at stake. This is a reality that should not be ignored.

Chapter 15: Why Decluttering the Mind Is Important Right Now

If you've read the rest of the chapters in this book thus far, then there is no reason why you should not be convinced that decluttering your mind is incredibly important; however, if you're thinking that decluttering the mind can wait until you're older, think again. Sure, you might be thinking that you're currently not in the right state of mind or are in the right circumstances to work towards this endeavour, but this chapter is here to convince you that eliminating mental clutter from your life is something that you should be seeking to do as soon as possible.

A Cluttered Mind Has Been Linked to Aging More Quickly

While you can certainly put off decluttering your mind until it works best for your lifestyle, you should be considering behaving in the opposite manner. Instead, you should be considering adapting your life to better promote a clear and stress-free brain. A major reason why this is so is that having too much going on in your brain in the form of stress, worrying, and anxiety has been directly linked to aging more quickly. Now, it would be counterproductive to worry about this. You don't need what this reality brings: even more clutter into your brain. However, that's not to say that you should not feel at least a little bit of urgency when it comes to finding a calmer state of mind for yourself.

Your Skin Needs Your Mind to Be Clear

For one, having more stress on the brain has been linked to actually speeding up the process that your cells go through from an aging perspective. You may not currently be aware of it, but your cells age just like you do. While the process itself is a tad complex, the point is that when your brain is being consumed by emotional distress, in particular, your skin cells actually begin to start maturing at a faster rate than they would if you were not experiencing these stressors. For this reason, it's best to keep the chapters in this book that were dedicated to discussing forming healthy relationships for yourself to heart. Otherwise, you're going to look in the mirror and feel as if you look like you're fifty when you're still thirty.

Stress and Sex

Another potentially more direct and detrimental by-product of worrying too much and thinking too much, in general, has to do with your sexual organs. Of course, the negative effects that too much mental clutter can have on your sex life is going to largely depend on whether you're a man or a woman. For men, it's possible for stress to cause a decrease in testosterone. This can lead to not just a decrease in your sperm count, but also potential problems associated with erectile dysfunction. It's safe to say that no one wants to have to deal with this type of problem if they don't have to.

On the other hand, if you're a woman and know that your mind is under a lot of stress, there's a chance that you could start experiencing problems related to your menstrual cycle. These problems can include irregularity of your period or extremely heavy periods that come with unpleasant and rather painful side effects. Having a period that is predictable and only mildly painful is always going to be preferable to a period that is so painful that you are unable to leave the house. Not only that, but an irregular period can be stressful in and of itself. When you don't know when to expect that type of monthly visit, it can influence your sexual relationships with your partner or can even lead to more stress because you end up worrying about whether your lack of a period is actually a pregnancy. For these reasons related to sex, it's best to try and eliminate mental clutter from your life now instead of later.

Mental Clutter Can Lead to a Greater Chance of a Stroke or Heart Attack

Not to sound too dismal, but if you want to decrease your chances of having a stroke or a heart attack, it's best to eliminate any stressful mental clutter from your life as quickly as possible. We already know that mental clutter can cause the sympathetic nervous system to start running (remember, your fight or flight response), but that's just one part of the body that gets moving more quickly when you've got a lot on your mind. For one thing, you begin to breathe more quickly when you're under stress. This means that if you already have asthma, mental clutter can exacerbate it.

In addition to breathing more quickly, mental clutter can also cause your heart to pump more quickly. We've all probably felt our heartbeat quicken when we're spending our time worrying about something that might be out of our control. If you allow your mind to do this often enough, know that you are putting a lot of stress on that heart of yours. You've only got one heart, and one way that you can honour the amazing things that your heart does is to go easy on it whenever you can. Not only that but when you have a lot on your mind and feel yourself becoming stressed, your body is releasing stress hormones.   When this happens, your stress hormones are being released as a way to provide your body's muscles with more oxygen so that you can take action more easily; however, at the same time, this is also increasing your blood pressure.   When the thoughts in your head are causing your body to raise its blood pressure on a consistent basis, this makes you more vulnerable to experiencing either a heart attack or a stroke.

If you're young, you might be reading this and thinking that these worries do not apply to you; however, you need to think about the fact that the habits that you cultivate when you're young will dictate how your body reacts to situations when you're older.   This is why it's important to take care of the beautiful body that you have now so that you don't start worrying about its well-being when it's too late.   It's that simple.   No one wants to be reliant on medication or therapy when they're older.   If you dedicate yourself to decluttering your brain now, rather than later, you're going to eventually look back one day and thank yourself for developing healthy and positive habits.

Conclusion

Congratulations on making it to the end of *Clear Your Mind: Regain Focus and Declutter Your Mental Space*. Hopefully, this book has been able to make you feel enlightened and more confident about how you can best navigate the inner workings of yourself. Often when the mind is cluttered, we can feel like we're all alone with no options. This book hopefully has been able to show you that you do have plenty of options when it comes to finding an inner balance and sense of calm. Understanding the concepts that were presented in this book is only the first step.

The next step towards creating a healthy internal environment involves starting small. Decide which area of your mind you're going to start working on first, and go from there. Implement some of the tactics that were presented in this book, and don't forget to be patient with yourself. Alteration of any type of habit, be it mental or physical, can often be a challenge. It's important to be steadfast in your pursuit of a clearer mind, but also realistic with yourself as well. The change will come in the smallest ways at first. It's important to appreciate and acknowledge these small victories when they do occur.

Lastly, if you enjoyed this book, *Clear Your Mind: Regain Focus and Declutter Your Mental Space,* a review on Amazon is always appreciated! Thank you.

Thank You

Please leave a review for this book online

Craig Crofts